PURE AMBROSIA

MONA LAJAUNIE
DUSTIN LAJAUNIE

CONTENTS

Introduction v

1. Mona's Main Dishes 1
2. Dustin's Main Dishes 26
3. Desserts 35

INTRODUCTION

From a very early age food played a special part in my life.

Food helped us celebrate, mourn, and reward achievements. We made traditional recipes to demonstrate love, affection, and appreciation. We shared our special dishes to signify acceptance into the family.

Until the age of 14, I lived in a small town in northern Mississippi. It was part of the Mississippi Delta, where rich, fertile soil has accumulated over eons of flooding and sediment settling onto the surrounding flood plains. Great for cotton. That was our reality. My dad was raised on a cotton plantation and his dad, my "Big Pop," was the overseer. It was a rough, lean existence. Those conditions, however, helped create strong familial bonds.

Many of my Dad's family — Edwin Parks (wife Helen and children Valorie and Sandra), Albert Lynwood Parks (wife Bonnie and children Bobbie and Carolynn) — lived there too.

Almost every weekend we would gather as a family to barbecue and/or have a fish fry.

The barbecue would consist of a homemade grill full of chicken, pork ribs, sausage, and on very rare occasions, t-bone steaks.

The side dishes were baked beans with hamburger meat and potato salad.

The fish fries were planned after all the men had returned from a fishing trip on the Mississippi River. The spread consisted of fried catfish (if they were female, the eggs would be taken and fried also), hushpuppies (my dad always claimed to make the best and everyone agreed), fresh cut french fries, and cole slaw.

However, this wasn't just about eating; It was about family, about survival, about wherewithal, about knowledge, about life, about love.

After the eating was done, we would move all the furniture in the living room, turn on the music, and dance and celebrate life. These good times lasted well into the night and were generally lubricated by lots of alcohol consumption by the adults.

My mother's family lived about 30 miles from my hometown.

I remember visiting my Mammaw (Jimmie Lucille Mathew Warren) and helping her churn butter and make butter molds.

We would gather vegetables from the garden and spend all day on the front porch rocking and visiting while shelling beans, cutting okra, and/or snapping green beans.

The clothes dryer was in the kitchen and was draped with a special guest towel. When Mammaw knew we were coming to visit, she would start to bake. The dryer displayed her labors of love. Carefully and lovingly placed on top were her famous pound cake and pecan pie. On the kitchen counter there was a tea kettle cookie jar filled with fresh baked cookies. On Sundays everyone went to church except my Mammaw; she would stay home to prepare lunch for the family.

When we returned from church the table was covered with fried chicken, mashed potatoes and gravy, fresh vegetables from the garden and either cornbread or biscuits. Everything made from scratch.

My mom must have molded herself after my Mammaw because she cooked three full-course meals a day. Always. Every day.

Breakfast mostly consisted of bacon or sausage, fried eggs over easy, grits, and biscuits with either red-eye gravy(made with ham dripping and coffee) or white gravy (made with sausage crumbles leftover with added flour and milk).

Lunch/dinner would have a meat (liver, chicken, pork chops, hamburger patties, etc), a vegetable, a starch and bread, and dessert.

The holidays were my mom's favorite time of the year. She would make several loaves of banana nut bread for the family and to share with friends. This was a tradition everyone looked forward to. On Christmas day we always had her amazing cornbread dressing with green bean and sweet potato casseroles among other dishes. On New Year's Eve she would prepare a huge pot of cabbage rolls for everybody.

At the age of 14, my dad moved us to Thibodaux, Louisiana.

Culture shock!

My dad was determined to "fit in" and began his journey of becoming a "transplant coonass." He was the occasional cook who loved watching Food Network shows and trying out-of-the-ordinary recipes.

He mastered the skill of boiling crawfish after many tries.

He made the best turnip stew, with pork and andouille sausage.

He assembled a turducken one Thanksgiving.

His Shrimp Mosca — named for the restaurant where he'd

first encountered the dish — was to-die-for!

His other cooking endeavors included: broiled oysters, red fish coubion, seafood gumbo, chicken and sausage gumbo, jambalaya. He succeeded in becoming a great "Cajun" cook.

And as the leader of our family, he inspired the rest of us, including my boys, to aspire to that same level of culinary mastery. (Along with an extremely high tolerance for alcohol. Facepalm.)

My desire is to create comfort foods; traditional foods that incubate and encourage and attract the same loving togetherness that we had in my family that wn still enjoy without compromising our health.

I have merely taken some of these very special meals and removed the meat, oils, dairy, refined flours and sugars. The love is all the same.

I am still showing my family love through food. It just looks a little different than Momma's cooking. Same labor of love, but in a healthier way. And, given what we have learned about health as a family, I think she's proud of my approach in the kitchen these days. I know she's watching.

From my family kitchen to yours, I hope you not only enjoy these healthier traditional meals —that were a huge part of my childhood and have since been handed down to my children — and enjoy them with loved ones gathered around the table, but use them as an opportunity to start exploring this new world of plant-based food, and what it can bring to the table for your family's health, in a new way.

I hope you hold on loosely to the directions, and free yourself to explore and be innovative. For *that* is the essence of what my family is about, the essence of what my parents seeded here in south Louisiana.

My son Dustin and I have put together some recipes that are either part of our regular lives or for our family gatherings these days. While they don't all resemble the old dishes of my and his youth, some do, and they all are life-giving instead of life-taking.

My mom and my dad, Dustin's "Mammaw and Bam Bam" gave their lives giving us what they thought was a leg-up on life and health and happiness through consumption: consumption of food; consumption of alcohol; consumption of health products, pills, procedures and hacks.

This was a very understandable misstep, given their depression-era upbringing. To be able to shower your family with boundless consumption must have felt right and good. And we love every memory we created along the way, even though we know now how that consumption-happy lifestyle contributed to their ultimate fate.

These foods, recipes, and dishes contributed to tragic losses in our lives: parents and siblings whose lives were cut short by heart disease; cousins who suffered and succumbed to the ravages of cancer; uncles and aunts whose vitality was erased by diabetes.

Even knowing that, though, it's still impossible for me to view these traditions as anything other than love and fond memories. When I first learned about the connection between processed foods and animal products and chronic disease, I felt torn. Throwing away these food traditions felt disloyal.

Eventually, I came to understand that some of the food I grew up with was actually survival food: what you ate when you didn't have other options. And some of our favorite daily meals had been once-a-year celebrations of bounty: when the yearling hog was butchered, or when the catfish eggs were harvested.

The real meaning of our food culture, I realized, was the dance between those extremes: survival and celebration.

So now I honor my ancestors' survival drive by making food that heals rather than harms. And I honor the celebratory nature of family gatherings by promoting our health and vigor with nutrient-rich meals that fuel our joyful expressions of life.

Instead of recreating the exact same meals that harmed us, I have decided to share those traditions and memories that show love, but with a different twist.

Showing love with food is not the problem. The type of food is the problem.

Let's make traditions, and show love with food that is healthy, filling, delicious, and forgiving if overeaten from time to time. We can still have some of those very special meals - they just require a little tweaking. We can still gather as a family and celebrate our proficiency at attaining sustenance that — ironic as it is to say— doesn't kill us slowly over time.

We present these recipes in a simple form on purpose. We want you to explore with us. Grow what you learn here. Apply the principles to morph your own food memories into live-giving, love-filled meals.

Now, let's get in the kitchen and rattle some pots n pans!

MONA'S MAIN DISHES

VEGGIE PASTALAYA

- 1 16-oz container Guidry's Creole Seasoning*
- 1 medium yellow squash (grated)
- 1 medium zucchini (grated)
- 1 8-oz container of mushrooms (chopped)
- 1 12-oz bag rotini pasta (cooked al dente)
- 2 tsp liquid smoke
- 2 tsp granulated garlic
- 2 tsp granulated onion
- ¼ tsp poultry seasoning
- 1 cup nutritional yeast
- ¼ cup tamari
- 2 ¼ cups vegetable broth, separated
- salt & pepper to taste

*Or DIY your own version of Guidry's:

- 1 cup chopped onions
- ½ cup chopped bell pepper
- ½ cup chopped celery
- ¼ cup fresh chopped parsley
- 1 tbsp minced garlic

INSTRUCTIONS

Cook Guidry's Creole Seasoning (or your DIY equivalent), squash, zucchini, and mushrooms in a stock pot on medium to high heat until everything begins to caramelize

Add 2 cups vegetable broth, liquid smoke, granulated garlic and onion, and poultry seasoning.

In a separate bowl combine 1 cup nutritional yeast, tamari,

and ¼ cup vegetable broth. Add to pot and stir. Add cooked pasta and mix everything together. Turn off , cover, and let set about 20 minutes before serving.

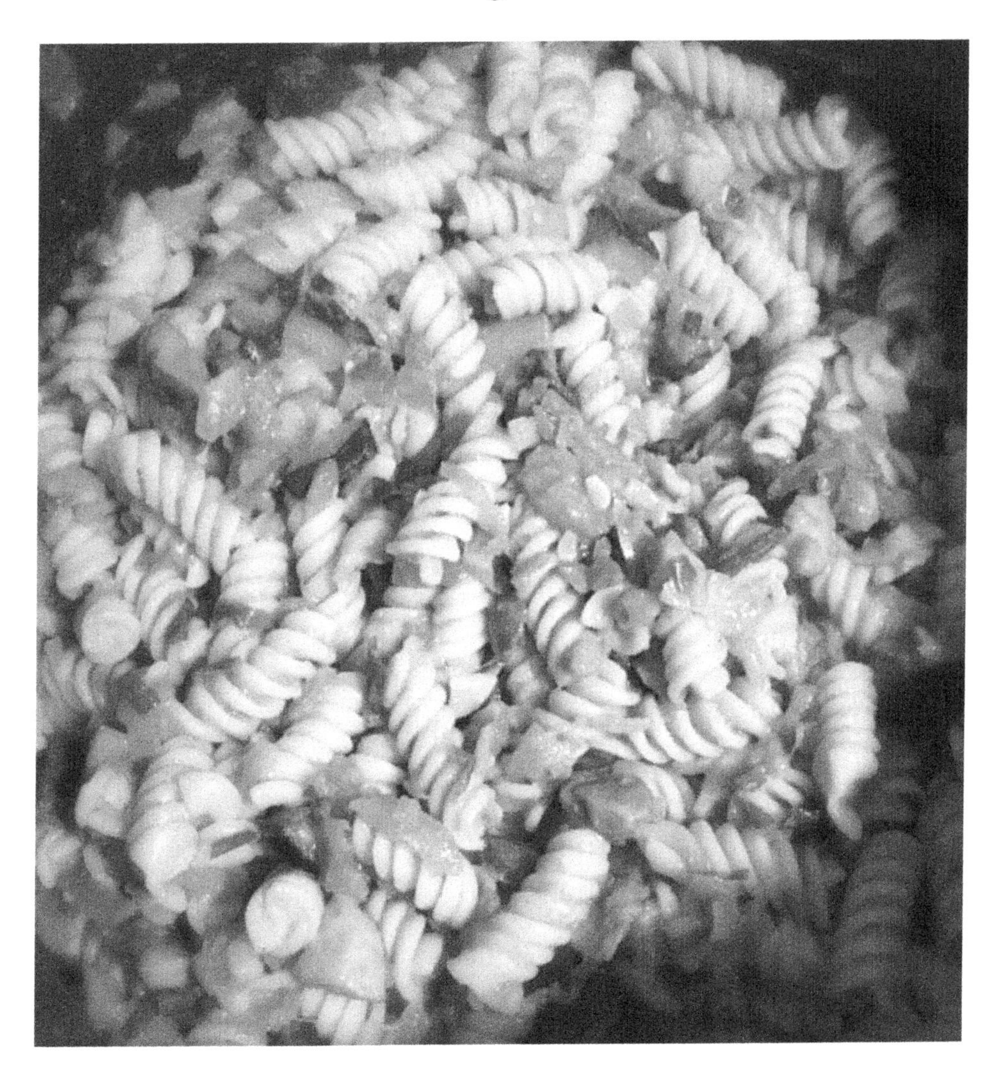

OKRA GUMBO

- 1 16-oz container Guidry's Creole Seasoning*
- 1 ½ cups oat flour (roux)
- 2 32-oz boxes of vegetable broth
- 1 to 2 can Rotel tomatoes and peppers (spicy)
- 1 family-size bag frozen cut okra (about 28oz)
- 2 tbsp liquid smoke
- 1 tbsp granulated garlic
- 1 tbsp granulated onion
- 1 tsp cayenne pepper
- ½ tsp poultry seasoning
- ½ cup nutritional yeast
- 6 cups water
- Salt & pepper to taste
- 4-6 cups cooked rice

*Or DIY your own version of Guidry's:

- 1 cup chopped onions
- ½ cup chopped bell pepper
- ½ cup chopped celery
- ¼ cup fresh chopped parsley
- 1 tbsp minced garlic

INSTRUCTIONS

Have Guidry's Creole Seasoning (or your DIY equivalent), vegetable broth, and water ready. (When the roux is done you will need to add these ingredients quickly.)

In large, heavy pot, cook oat flour (roux) over medium to high heat stirring constantly. (This can burn quickly. Be vigilant).

When the flour is a little darker than the color of peanut butter add chopped creole seasoning and stir briefly to coat.

Add both boxes of vegetable broth. The liquid will begin to thicken. Stir as the liquid thickens, and pour in the water.

Add cayenne pepper, granulated garlic/onion, poultry seasoning, liquid smoke, nutritional yeast, Rotel, and frozen okra.

Simmer for 1 ½ to 2 hours (the longer the better). Stir as needed to prevent burning on the bottom. Season to taste with salt and pepper. Serve over rice.

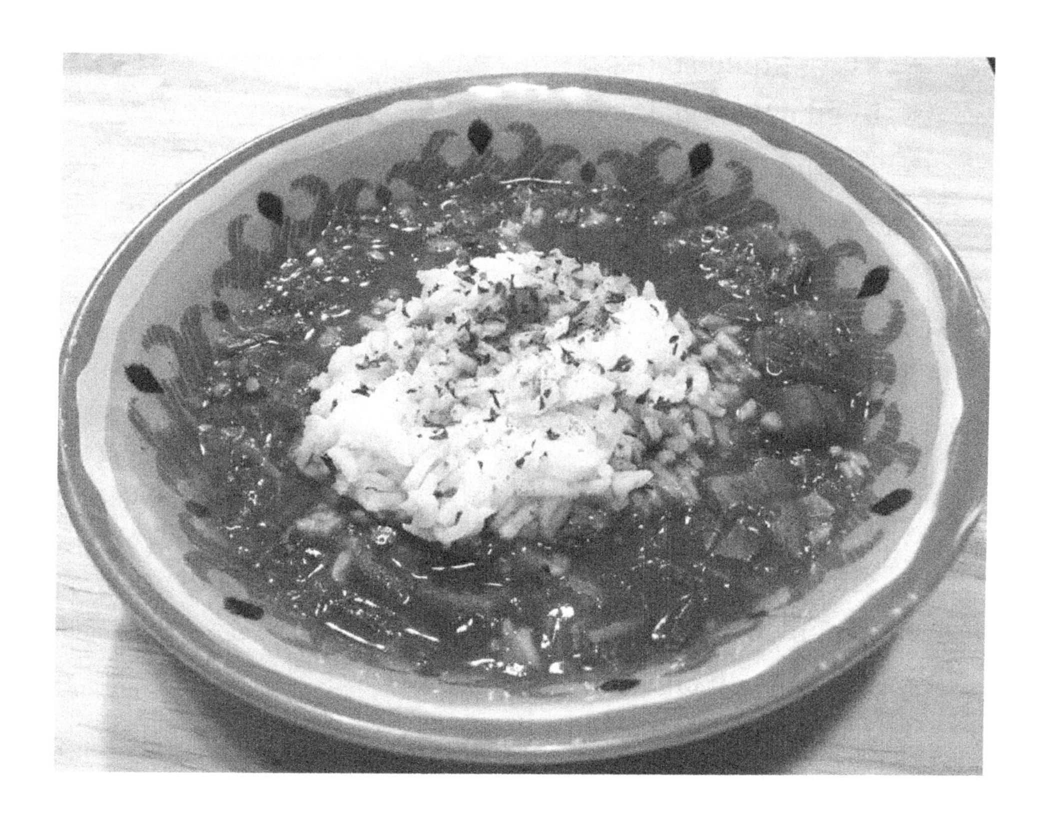

MOMMA'S VEGGIE JAMBALAYA

- 1 16-oz container Guidry's Creole Seasoning*
- 4 ¾ cups vegetable broth
- 2 medium zucchini (chopped)
- 1 medium squash (chopped)
- 1 8-oz container of sliced mushrooms
- 2 medium carrots (shredded)
- 6 green onions (chopped)
- 1 tsp granulated garlic
- 1 tsp granulated onion
- 1 tbsp liquid smoke
- 1 cup nutritional yeast
- ¼ cup water
- ¼ cup tamari
- ⅛ tsp poultry seasoning
- Salt & pepper to taste
- 3 cups rice

*Or DIY your own version of Guidry's:

- 1 cup chopped onions
- ½ cup chopped bell pepper
- ½ cup chopped celery
- ¼ cup fresh chopped parsley
- 1 tbsp minced garlic

INSTRUCTIONS

In stock pot, sauté chopped creole seasoning (or your DIY equivalent), zucchini, squash, carrot, and mushrooms on medium heat.

When the veggies begin to stick to the bottom, add a scant amount of water and continue cooking until caramelized. Watch closely and stir often: this process takes 30-45 minutes.

In a separate bowl, mix together nutritional yeast, tamari, and water. Add this mixture to the stock pot once the vegetables are caramelized.

Add vegetable broth, liquid smoke, poultry seasoning, granulated garlic/onion, salt/pepper to taste, and bring to boil.

Add green onions and rice, and stir to mix evenly.

Cover and simmer on low heat for 20-30 minutes, stirring occasionally, until the liquid is absorbed.

Keeping the lid on, remove from heat and let set 15-20 minutes before serving.

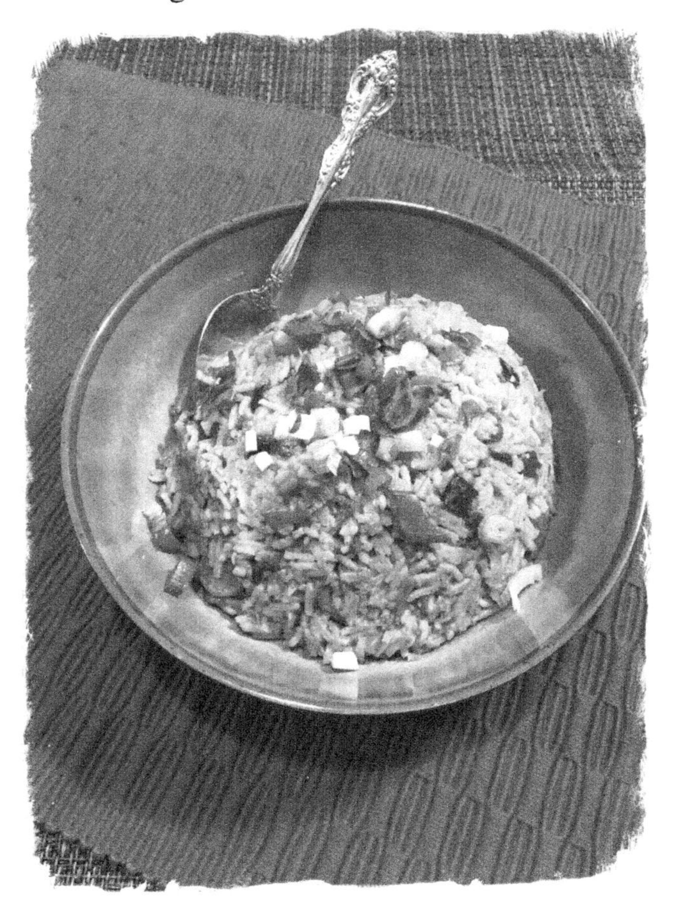

MEENIE'S BBQ LENTIL LOAF

- 1 16-oz container Guidry's Creole Seasoning*
- 1 8-oz container mushrooms chopped
- 6 cups cooked red lentils
- 1 tbsp granulated garlic
- 1 tbsp granulated onion
- ⅓ cup tamari
- 1 ½ tbsp liquid smoke
- ½ cup nutritional yeast
- 1 cup oat flour
- 1 cup rolled oats
- ½ cup BBQ sauce
- 2 cups brown rice

*Or DIY your own version of Guidry's:

- 1 cup chopped onions
- ½ cup chopped bell pepper
- ½ cup chopped celery
- ¼ cup fresh chopped parsley
- 1 tbsp minced garlic

INSTRUCTIONS

Sauté chopped creole seasoning (or your DIY equivalent) and mushrooms until tender.

In large bowl, combine sautéed mixture with remaining ingredients. Mix well.

If the mixture is too runny, add bread crumbs or more oat flour.

For best results, let the mixture sit in your fridge overnight.

If you can't wait that long, proceed to the next step as soon as the mixture is the consistency of cookie dough.

Place in two loaf pans. Bake at 350º F (180º C) for about 1 to 1 ½ hours.

Let set for 30 minutes to 1 hour before serving. It's even better the next day.

Meatball Option: Roll into balls and bake on a parchment-paper lined baking sheet for 25-30 minutes.

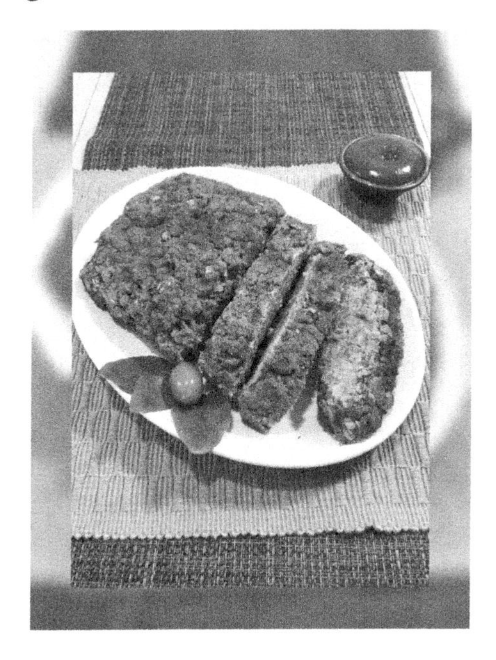

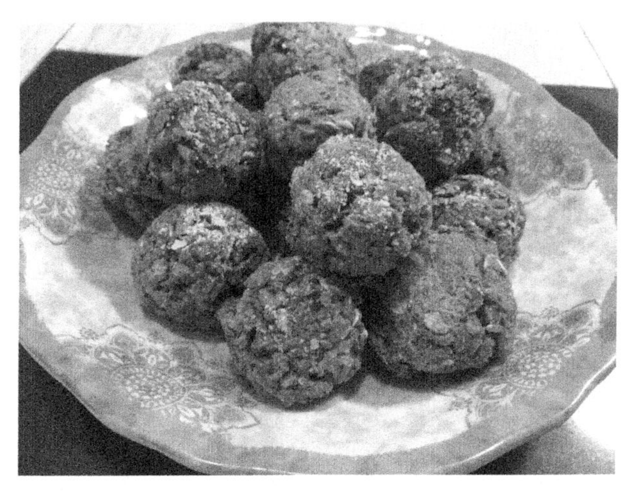

OATMEAL CASSEROLE

- 2 cups rolled oats
- ¼ cup raisins
- ¼ cup walnuts
- ½ cup blueberries (frozen)
- 2 tsp cinnamon
- 3 tbsp maple syrup
- ⅛ tsp vanilla extract
- Dash of salt
- 1 ¾ to 2 cups non-dairy milk (almond or coconut, unsweetened)
- 1 medium to large over-ripe banana, mashed

INSTRUCTIONS

Combine all ingredients in oven-safe casserole dish and mix well.

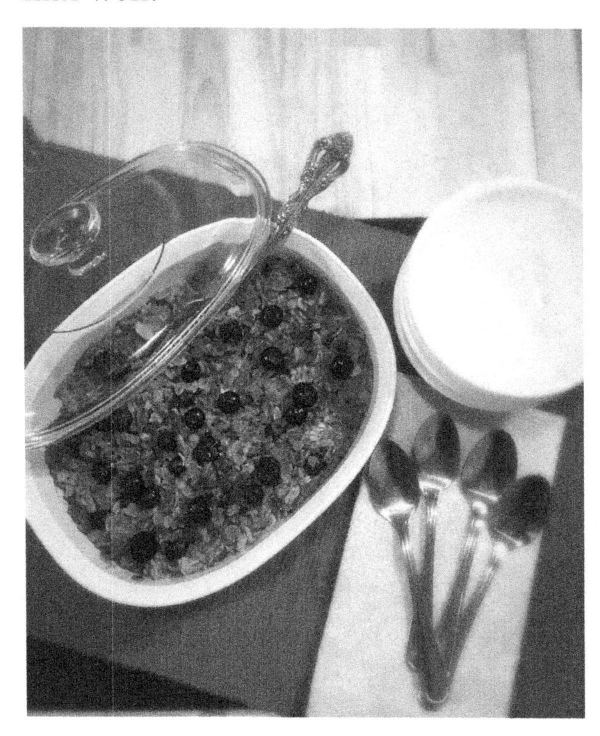

OVEN: Cover with a lid or aluminum foil, and bake at 350° F (180° C) for 30-45 minutes.

MICROWAVE: Cook for 4 minutes. Remove from microwave, stir and return to cook for another 3-4 minutes.

POTATO CORN CHOWDER

- 4 large potatoes (cubed)
- 2 15-oz cans whole kernel corn
- 1 medium onion (chopped)
- 3 large carrots (cubed or sliced with mandoline slicer)
- 1 ½ tsp granulated garlic
- 1 ½ tsp granulated onion
- 3-4 quarts water
- ¼ cup unsweetened almond milk
- salt/pepper to taste

INSTRUCTIONS

Place one can of corn in blender with ¼ cup unsweetened almond milk and blend slightly (consistency of cream corn) and set aside.

In medium to large pot place cubed potatoes and water (enough to cover potatoes by one inch). Boil until barely tender.

Add remaining ingredients (including blended corn) and cook until vegetables are tender (add water if needed). Stir as needed.

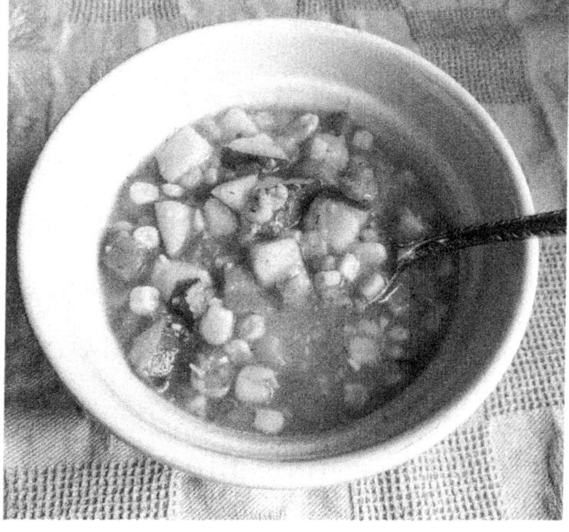

CHICKPEA NUGGETS

NUGGETS

- 1 15-oz can organic chickpeas
- ½ cup oat flour
- 1 tbsp Dijon mustard
- 1 tsp granulated garlic
- 1 tsp granulated onion
- ½ tsp salt
- ⅛ tsp poultry seasoning
- 3 tbsp water
- 1 tbsp nutritional yeast

COATING

- 1 to 1 ½ cups organic bread crumbs
- ¼ cup nutritional yeast
- ½ tsp granulated garlic
- ½ tsp granulated onion
- ¼ tsp salt

MILK WASH

- ½ cup almond milk

INSTRUCTIONS

Place parchment paper on cookie sheet.

In a bowl, mash chickpeas with a fork until smooth. Mix in remaining nugget ingredients and mix well.

Prepare coating by mixing all coating ingredients in a bowl. Set aside.

Put ½ cup of almond milk in separate bowl. Use small

cookie scoop to scoop nugget mixture and form into desired shape (one scoop = one nugget).

Dip nugget in almond milk and then roll in coating, making sure to cover completely. Place on cookie sheet. Continue until all mixture is used.

Bake in oven at 350° F (180° C) for about 15-20 minutes on each side, or until golden brown.

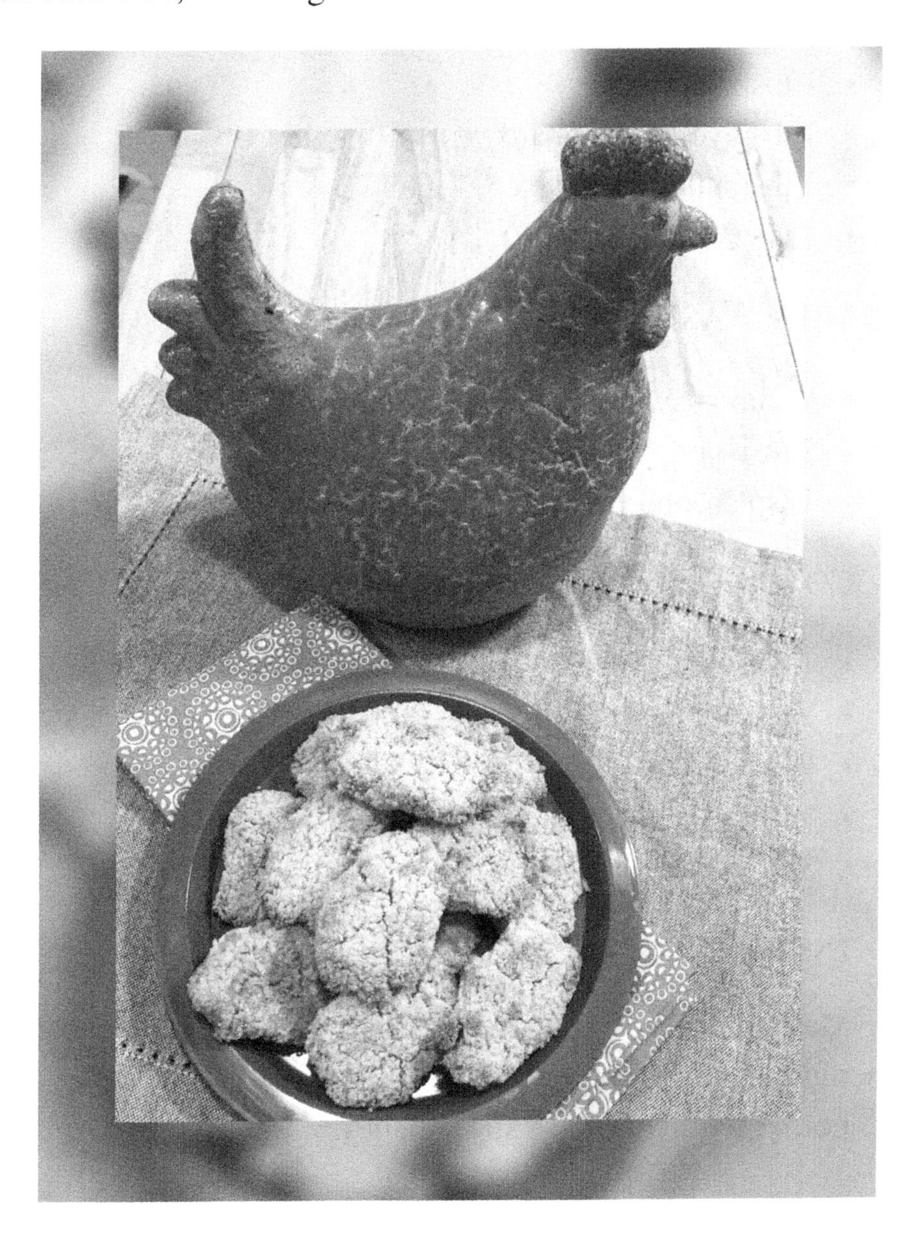

FISHLESS STICKS

STICKS

- 2 medium to large white potatoes (baked)
- ¾ cooked rice
- 1 tsp granulated garlic
- 1 tsp granulated onion
- 1 tsp salt (or to taste)
- 1 tbsp tahini
- 1 tbsp yellow mustard
- 1 tbsp nutritional yeast
- 2 tbsp corn flour

MILK WASH

- ¾ cup unsweetened almond milk
- 2 tbsp yellow mustard
- 1 tsp ground flax

COATING

- 1 cup organic bread crumbs
- ½ cup corn meal
- ½ tsp granulated garlic
- ½ tsp granulate onion
- Salt to taste

INSTRUCTIONS

Mash the baked potatoes in a large bowl. Add remaining stick ingredients and mix well.

Form mixture into fish stick shapes.

Dip in milk wash and roll in coating, making sure to cover each stick completely.

Place sticks on cookie sheet covered with parchment paper. Bake at 350 for about 15-20 minutes on each side or until golden brown.

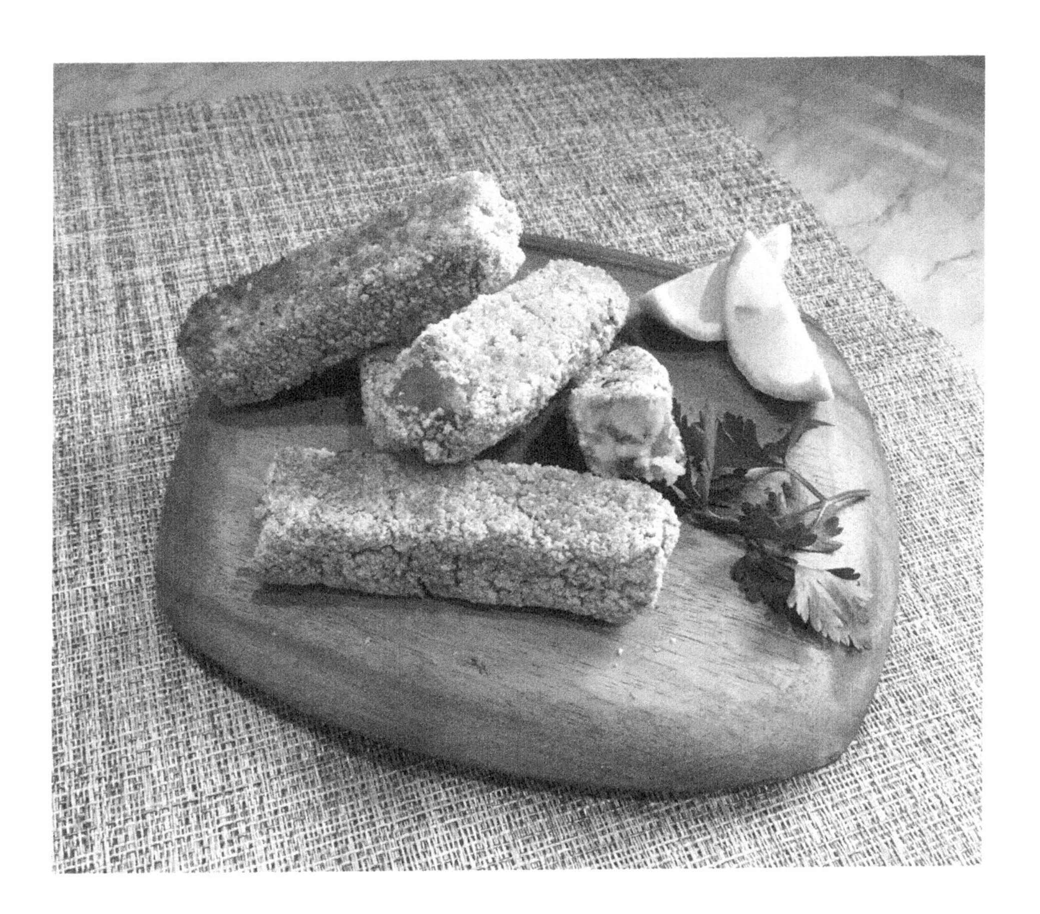

STUFFED BELL PEPPER

- 6 large bell peppers
- 3-4 eggplants (cubed)
- 1 large onion (chopped)
- 1 packet vegan brown gravy mix
- 1 ½ tsp granulated garlic
- 1 ½ tsp granulated onion
- 1 8-oz container mushrooms
- 1 ¼ cup cauliflower rice
- 1 cup chopped walnuts
- 3 ½ cups cooked rice
- ¾ cup organic bread crumbs
- ½ tsp cayenne pepper
- Salt & pepper to taste

INSTRUCTIONS

Place eggplant and onions in pan and sauté until tender (about 30-45 minutes). Turn off and set aside.

Place mushrooms in food processor and blend until fine. Place in separate pan. Add vegan brown gravy mix and cook about 20 minutes.

In the meantime, place cauliflower rice and walnuts in food processor and blend until fine. Add to pan and continue to cook about 20 more minutes.

Add mushroom mixture to eggplant and cook about 10-15 minutes. Add rice, ½ cup bread crumbs and all seasonings, and mix well.

Cut tops off bell pepper and remove seeds. Place eggplant/ mushroom mixture into bell pepper. Cover tops with remaining bread crumbs. Place bell pepper in cake pan with about ½ inch water. Bake at 350° F (180° C) for about 45 minutes to an hour (until bell pepper is tender).

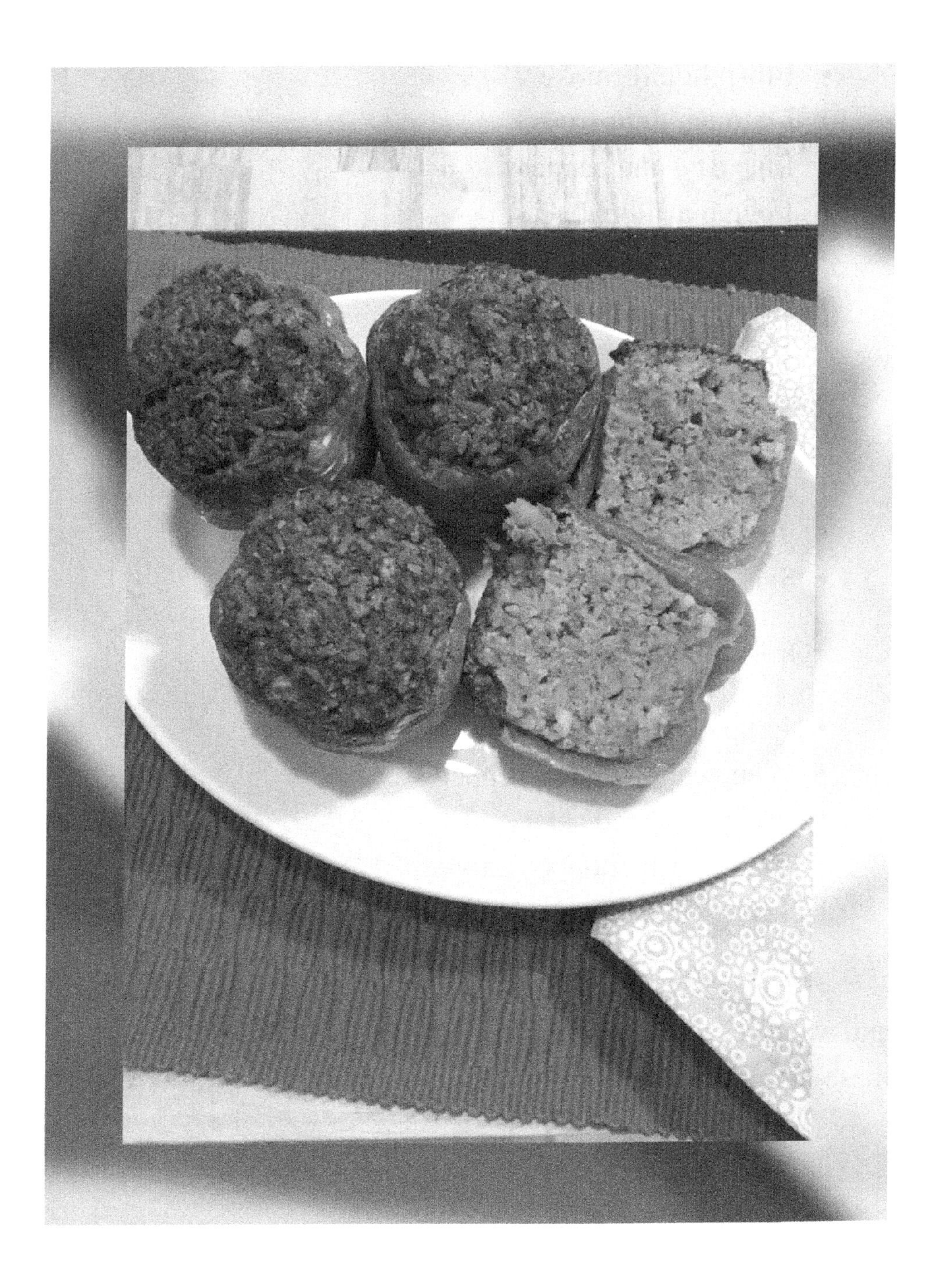

TURNIP STEW

- 1 16-oz container Guidry's Creole Seasoning*
- 1 tbsp granulated garlic
- 1 tbsp granulated onion
- 1 tbsp liquid smoke
- 1 cup oat flour (roux)
- 1 tsp cayenne pepper
- 1 cup nutritional yeast
- ¼ cup whole wheat flour
- 2 tbsp corn starch
- ¼ cup tamari
- 2 8-oz containers of sliced mushrooms
- 2 32-oz boxes of vegetable broth
- 2 ½ cups water
- 9-12 large turnips (cubed)
- Salt & pepper to taste

*Or DIY your own version of Guidry's:

- 1 cup chopped onions
- ½ cup chopped bell pepper
- ½ cup chopped celery
- ¼ cup fresh chopped parsley
- 1 tbsp minced garlic

**NOTE: Have chopped creole seasoning, vegetable broth and water ready. When the roux is done you will need to add these ingredients quickly.

INSTRUCTIONS

Have Guidry's Creole Seasoning (or your DIY equivalent), vegetable broth, and water ready. (When the roux is done you will need to add these ingredients quickly.)

In large, heavy pot, cook oat flour (roux) over medium to high heat stirring constantly. (This can burn quickly. Be vigilant).

When the flour is a little darker than the color of peanut butter add chopped creole seasoning and stir briefly to coat.

Stir as the liquid thickens, and pour in the water.

Add cayenne pepper, granulated garlic and onion, and liquid smoke. In a separate bowl, mix together nutritional yeast, tamari, and ½ cup water. Add to pot, stir and bring to boil.

Add mushrooms and turnips and bring the stew back to boil. Reduce heat, and simmer until turnips are tender (about 1 ½ hours), stirring as needed.

Season to taste with salt and pepper.

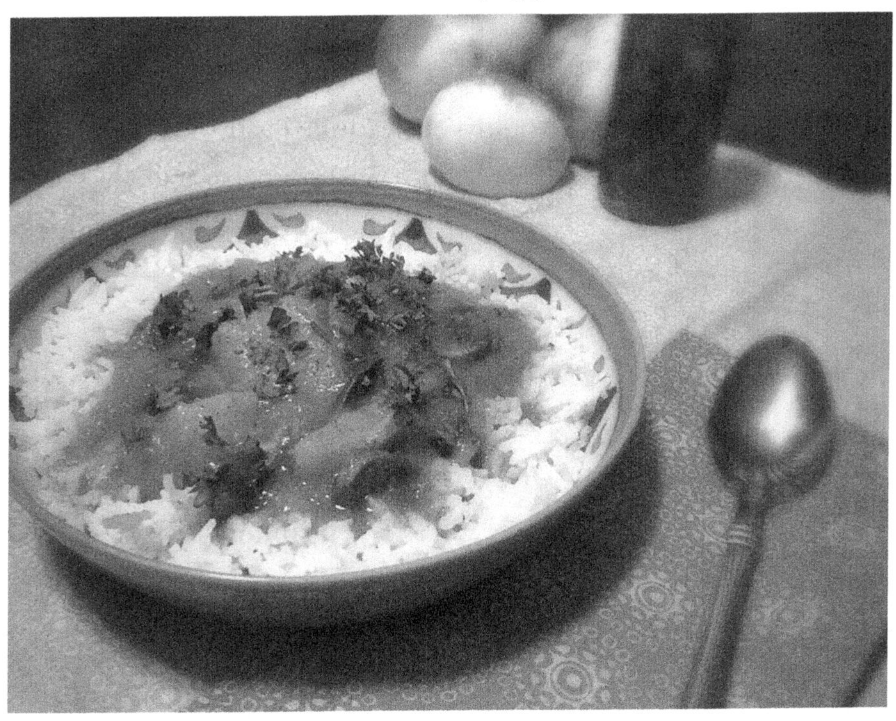

MUSHROOM RICE

- 2 bags frozen brown rice
- 2 bags frozen pic sweet seasoning (onions and peppers)
- 2 8-oz containers of button mushrooms (sliced thin)
- 1 bag frozen sliced carrots
- 2 medium potatoes (cubed)
- 1 cup nutritional yeast
- ¼ cup tamari
- ¼ cup water
- 1 tsp granulated garlic
- 1 tsp granulated onion
- ½ tsp cayenne pepper
- ½ tsp crushed red pepper flakes
- salt/pepper to taste

INSTRUCTIONS

In a bowl, mix nutritional yeast, tamari, and water. Set aside.

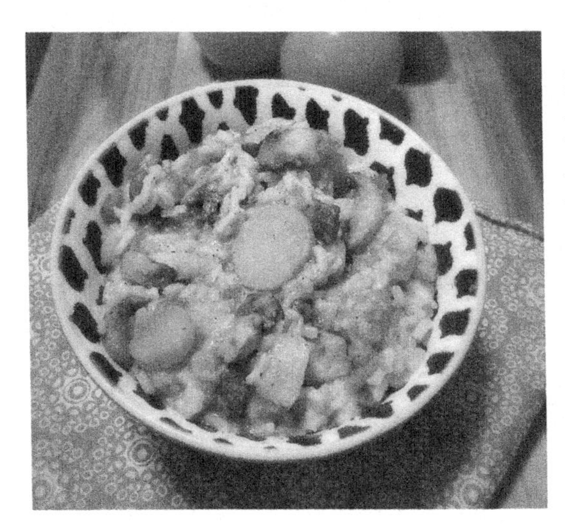

Throw all remaining ingredients in an Instant Pot or other electric pressure cooker and add nutritional yeast mixture. Cook on high pressure for 13 minutes.

MITA'S VEGETABLE SOUP

- 1 small head of cabbage, chopped
- 2 medium onions, chopped
- 3 large potatoes, cut into chunks
- 8 large carrots, cubed
- 1 32-oz box veggie broth
- 2 15-oz cans tomato sauce
- 1 bag frozen mixed vegetables (corn, green beans, carrots, peas)
- 8 cups water
- 2 tsp liquid smoke
- 1/3 cup minced garlic
- 2 cups nutritional yeast
- 2 tbsp garlic powder
- Salt/pepper to taste
- Louisiana Hot Sauce to taste

INSTRUCTIONS

Add cabbage, broth, and water to large pot, boil for 10 minutes, and add potatoes.

Cover and lower heat to medium, and cook for 15 minutes.

Add frozen vegetables, garlic powder, liquid smoke, nutritional yeast, and tomato sauce. Simmer for about 5 minutes, then add onions, garlic, and carrots.

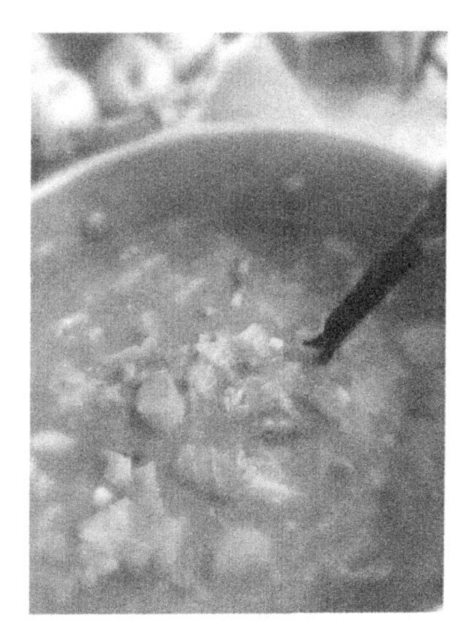

Simmer on low to medium heat for about 45 minutes, or until veggies are tender. Stir occasionally, taking care not to break the potatoes.

CABBAGE ROLLS

STUFFING

- 1 16-oz container Guidry's Creole Seasoning*
- 1 8-oz container mushrooms chopped
- 6 cups cooked red lentils
- 1 tbsp granulated garlic
- 1 tbsp granulated onion
- 1 ½ tsp cinnamon
- ⅓ cup tamari
- 1 ½ tbsp liquid smoke
- ½ cup nutritional yeast
- 1 cup oat flour
- 1 cup rolled oats
- 2 ½ cups brown or basmati rice
- 1 large onion (sliced)
- 2 15-oz cans of diced tomatoes

*Or DIY your own version of Guidry's:

- 1 cup chopped onions
- ½ cup chopped bell pepper
- ½ cup chopped celery
- ¼ cup fresh chopped parsley
- 1 tbsp minced garlic

CABBAGE

- 1-2 heads of cabbage
- 1 large onion (sliced)
- 2 15-oz cans of diced tomatoes
- salt and pepper to taste

INSTRUCTIONS

Sauté chopped creole seasoning (or your DIY equivalent) and mushrooms until tender.

In large bowl, add sautéed mixture and remaining ingredients with exception of cabbage, onion, and tomatoes. Mix well, and set aside.

Prepare cabbage: Cut out core. Place cabbage in pan with about an inch of water with core side down. Steam on high heat. When leaves begin to soften, peel off one at a time and set aside.

Prepare rolls: Take cabbage leaf, put in stuffing, roll cabbage leaf and secure with toothpick. (I fold both ends and then roll). Place cabbage rolls in large pot.

Add sliced onions, tomatoes, salt/pepper to taste. Cook until onions and tomatoes are tender.

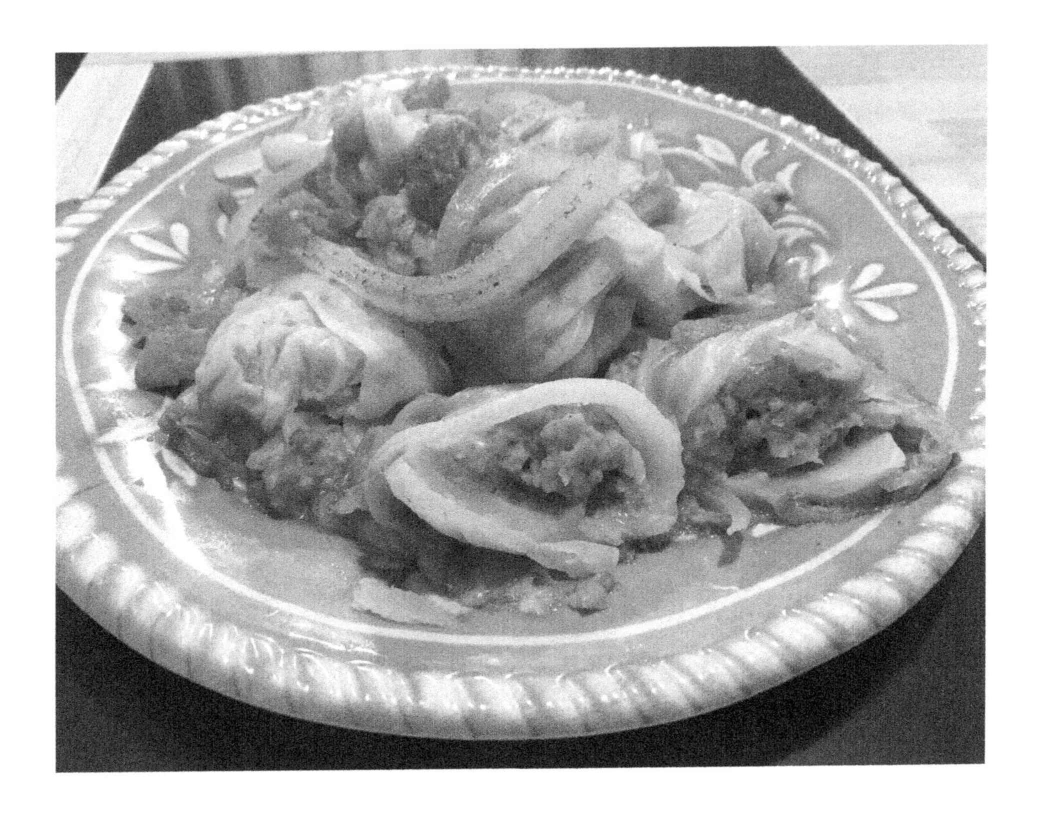

BEANS AND RICE

- 1 lb red or white dry beans (I use Blue Runner brand)
- 10-12 cups water
- 2 tbsp granulated garlic
- 2 tbsp granulate onion
- 2 tbsp liquid smoke
- 1 tbsp minced garlic
- 2 tbsp parsley flakes
- salt/pepper to taste
- 1 16-oz container Guidry's Creole Seasoning*
- 5-6 cups cooked rice

*Or DIY your own version of Guidry's:

- 1 cup chopped onions
- ½ cup chopped bell pepper
- ½ cup chopped celery
- ¼ cup fresh chopped parsley
- 1 tbsp minced garlic

INSTRUCTIONS

Soak beans in about 6-8 cups water for 2-4 hours (overnight is even better). Drain and place in a stock pot.

Add about 4-6 cups water (or vegetable broth) or enough liquid to cover beans about 1 inch). Bring to boil, turn heat to medium/low and let cook for about 1 hour.

Add granulated garlic/onion, liquid smoke, parsley flakes, minced garlic, salt/pepper, and creole seasoning. Turn heat to low.

Simmer (low and slow) for about 4 hours. The longer it simmers, the creamier it will be. To serve, place ¾ cup of rice in a bowl and cover it with beans.

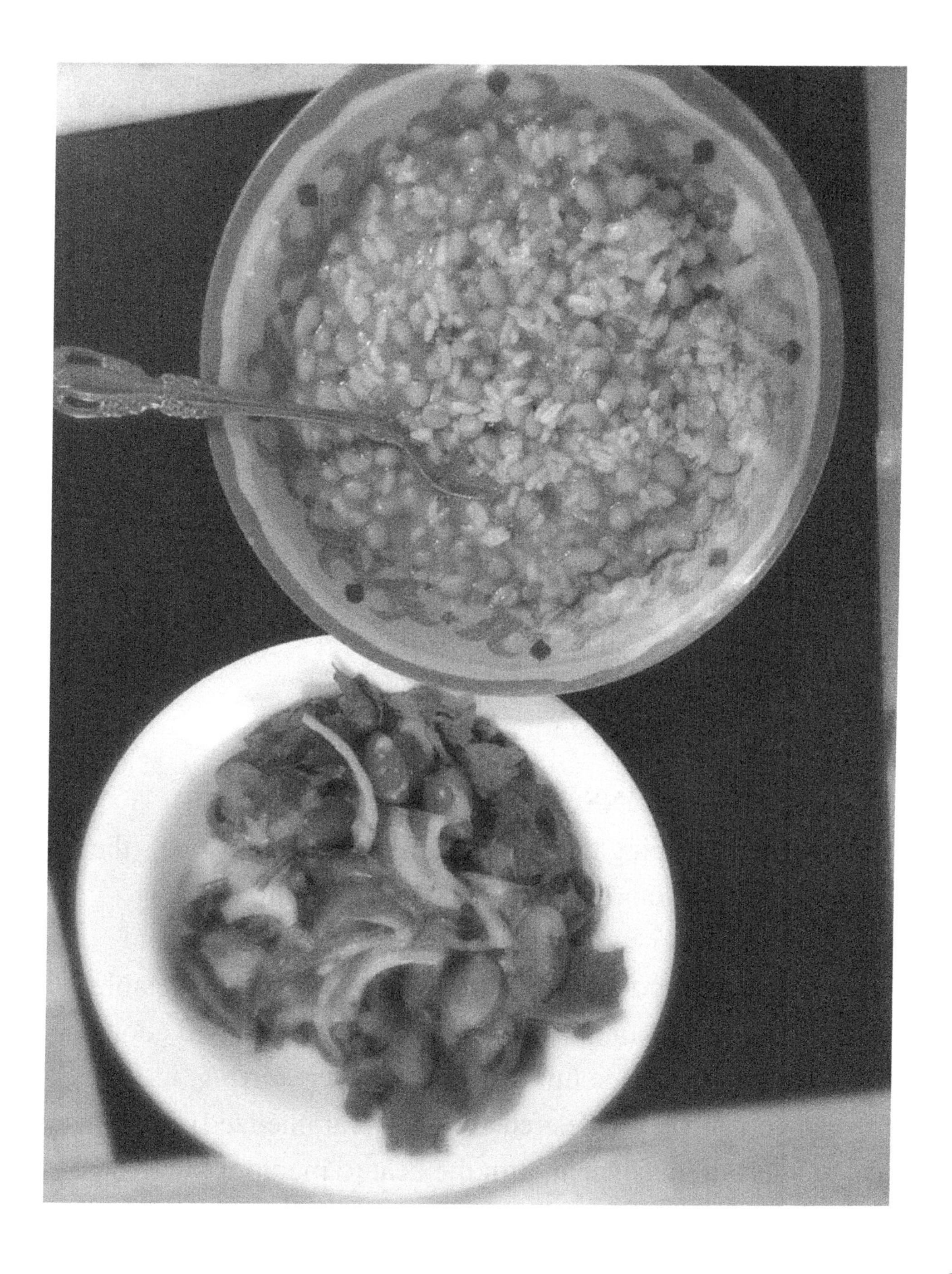

DUSTIN'S MAIN DISHES

Dustin's Jambalaya

- 2 cups onions (diced)
- 1 cup celery (diced)
- 1 cup bell pepper (diced)
- 2 cups mushrooms (diced)
- 1 cup tomatoes (diced)
- ⅔ cup green onions (chopped)
- ¼ cup minced garlic
- ⅓ cup tamari
- 7 cups vegetable broth (includes broth for deglazing)
- 3 tbsp liquid smoke
- 4 cups rice
- ½ cup nutritional yeast (nooch)
- ½ tsp cayenne pepper
- salt/pepper to taste

INSTRUCTIONS

Begin by placing the onions, celery, and bell pepper (the "trinity") in a large pot, keeping it on medium/high heat.

We want to encourage a little "burning" for flavor and color. Don't let it go too far without deglazing with vegetable broth. Use scant amounts of broth at a time or you will cool down the pot. Continue this process and keep stirring.

Once you get the desired "brown" (caramelized) color and onions are translucent, turn the heat to medium/low. Add mushrooms, tomatoes, and garlic. Allow to cook together for a few minutes.

Add tamari, liquid smoke, nooch, cayenne pepper, and salt/pepper to taste. Mix together and allow to cook down for about 10-15 minutes.

Now add rice. Stir well so rice is completely covered with the base. Add the remaining vegetable broth and stir well and bring to simmer for 10 minutes.

Turn heat to lowest setting and add green onions. Cover the pot and let cook for 10 minutes (do not uncover or stir). Turn off heat.

Uncover, fold over rice to move rice at the bottom to the top and vice-versa. Do this step quickly so not to lose too much steam.

Cover for another 10 minutes. Uncover again and stir using the previous method. Cover and let sit for another 10 minutes then serve. ENJOY!

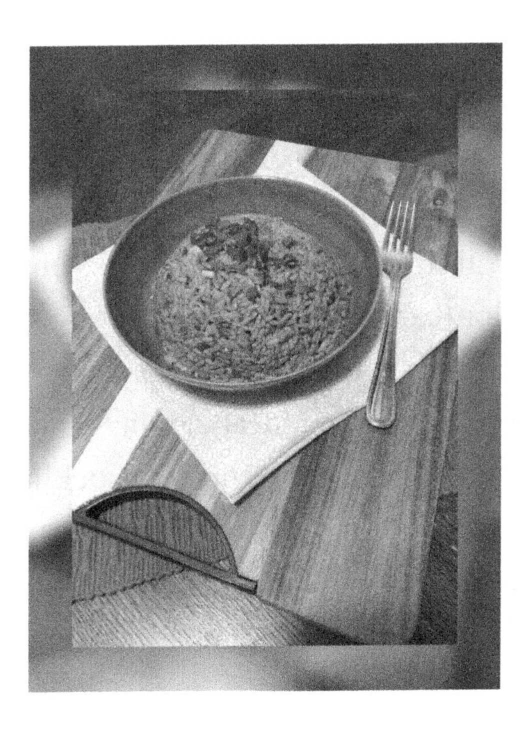

SAUCE PICANTE

- 3 cups onions (diced)
- 1 cup celery (diced)
- 1 cup bell pepper (diced)
- 2 cups tomatoes (diced)
- 2 8-oz cans tomato sauce
- 1 ½ cups mushrooms (sliced)
- ¼ cup minced garlic
- 1 cup green onions (chopped)
- 1 jalapeño pepper (finely chopped)
- 1 tsp cayenne pepper
- 2 tsp liquid smoke
- ½ cup nutritional yeast (nooch)
- Water or veggie broth for deglazing
- Salt/pepper to taste
- Cooked rice

INSTRUCTIONS

Place onions, celery, and bell peppers in a pot on medium-high heat. Let almost "burn" then add scant amount of water/veggie broth to deglaze. Continue this process until you have a golden brown color (caramelized).

Add tomatoes, mushrooms, jalapeño pepper, garlic, and green onions. Cook on medium heat, adding scant amount of water or veggie broth as needed to prevent sticking.

Simmer with lid on for about 30 minutes, stirring as needed. Add cayenne pepper, liquid smoke, and nooch. Cook on medium-low heat for another 30 minutes, stirring occasionally.

Add lemon juice and turn to low heat. Cook for another 10-15 minutes. Remove from heat. Add salt and pepper to taste. Serve over cooked rice.

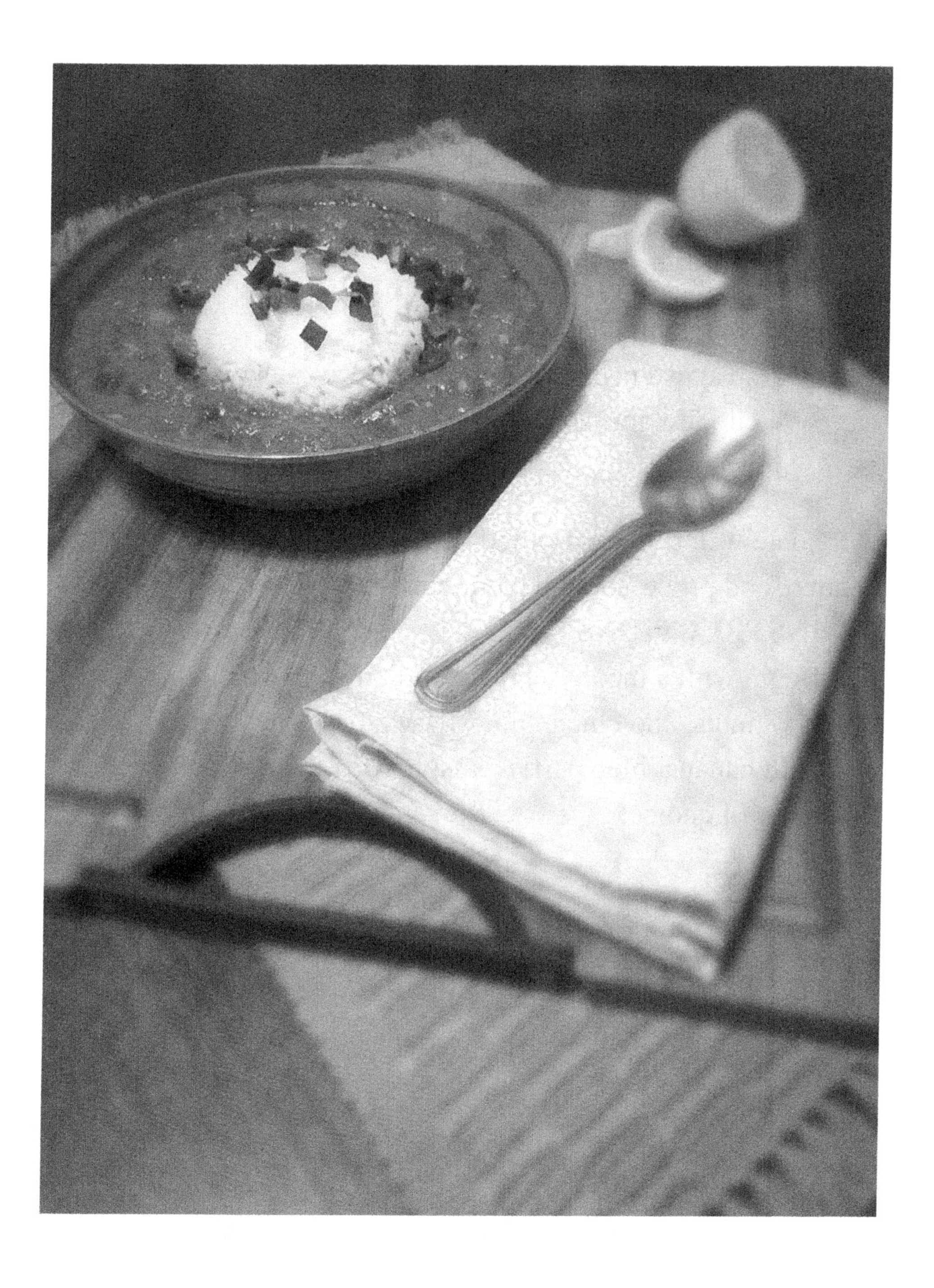

DYNAMIC BREAKFAST BOWL

- ¾ cup oats
- 1 tsp ground flax
- 1 tsp hemp hearts
- 2 tbsp walnuts (chopped)
- 1 banana (sliced or chopped)
- ¼ cup blueberries (fresh or frozen)
- ¼ cup raspberries (fresh or frozen)
- cinnamon to taste
- ¼ tsp lemon juice
- 1 tsp agave nectar or maple syrup, or date water*
- ¾ cup flax milk (can substitute any plant-based milk)

*date water: place 1 pitted date and 1 cup of water in blender/food processor and blend well.

INSTRUCTIONS

Begin with a medium bowl. Add oats, ground flax, hemp hearts, walnuts, and cinnamon. Mix well.

Add banana, blue berries, raspberries, lemon juice, and sweetener of choice.

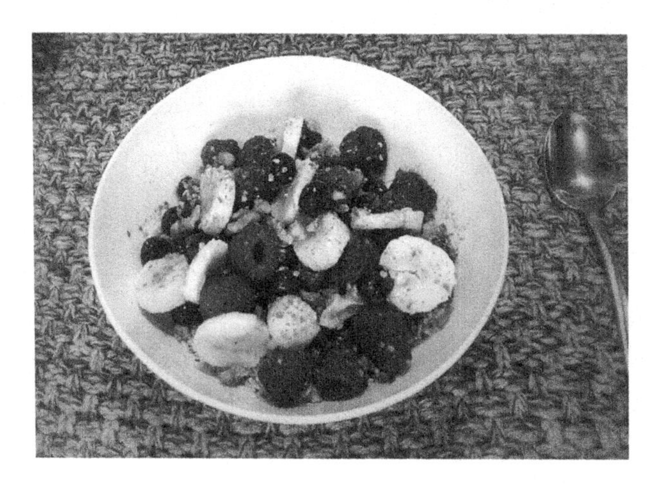

HEAVENLY HASH BROWNS

- 6 medium potatoes (diced)
- 1 onion (julienne)
- 1 bell pepper (julienne)
- 1 tsp granulated garlic
- 1 cup mushrooms (sliced)
- ½ cup green onions (chopped)
- Salt/pepper to taste

INSTRUCTIONS

Preheat oven to 475° F (250° C). Place diced potatoes on cookie sheet and spread evenly. Cook in oven for 10-15 minutes.

While potatoes are cooking, get a large skillet, add a small amount of water (about 1-2 tsp) and place on medium-high heat. Add onions, bell pepper, and mushrooms, and cook briefly until transparent. Check potatoes, take out of oven, flip them over and place back into oven until golden brown.

When potatoes are done, take them out and place in skillet with onions, bell peppers, and mushrooms. Add granulated garlic and salt/pepper to taste. Allow to cook on low-medium heat until tender. Remove from heat and let cool about 10 minutes before serving.

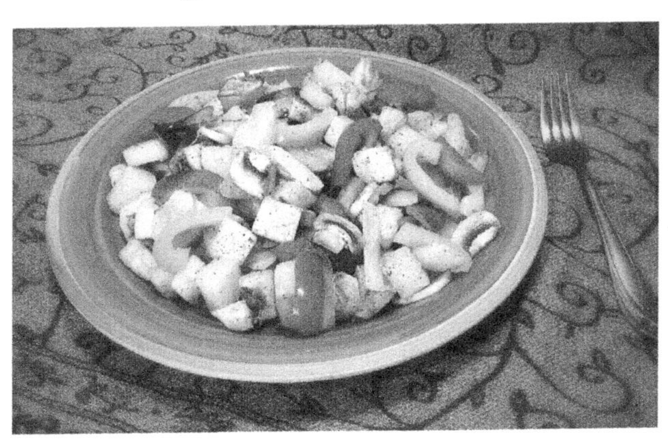

VEGGIE KABOBS AND TATER SLABS

- 2 onions (cut into 1" chunks)
- 2 bell peppers (cut into 1" chunks)
- 1 package cherry tomatoes (whole)
- 1 package whole mushrooms
- 2 -yellow squash (cut into 1/2" thick slices)
- 2 zucchini (cut into 1/2" thick slices)
- 1 tbsp minced garlic
- 1 large baking potato (cut full length into ½" thick slabs)
- 10 wooden skewers
- granulated garlic
- salt/pepper to taste

INSTRUCTIONS

Begin by soaking the wooden skewers in water while you prep the veggies.

Place prepped onions, bell peppers, squash, zucchini, mushrooms, tomatoes in bowl. Add the minced garlic and salt/pepper to taste. Mix well so all veggies are covered with seasoning and let set.

Lay the potato slabs on a cookie sheet and season with granulated garlic and salt/pepper to taste.

Now begin building your veggie kabobs. Place veggies on skewer in random order, being careful not to use same veggie twice in a row. This will give you colorful and flavorful kabobs.

It's time to light the pit (medium temperature). When pit is ready, place the potato slabs on the grill (not over direct flame). They will stick at first but then will begin to crust over. Now place the veggie kabobs on the grill and cook until desired tenderness.

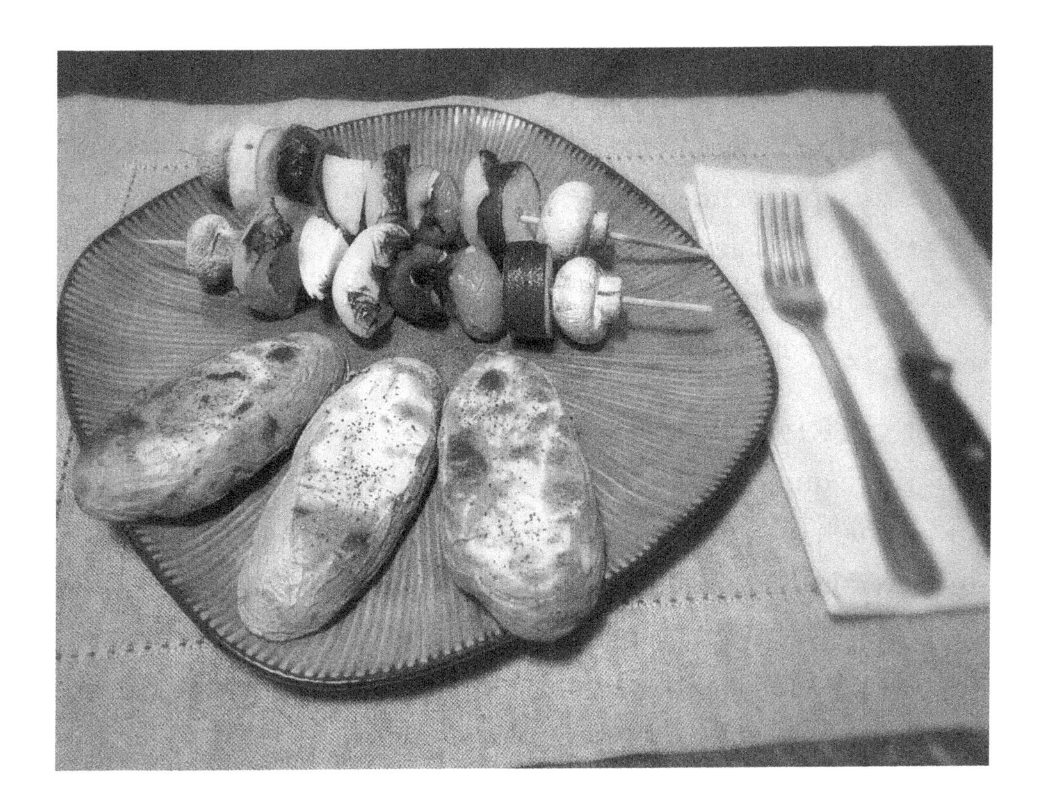

MEXI-ANA QUINOA SALAD

- 2 cups dry quinoa
- ½ cup purple/red onion (chopped)
- 1 large tomato (diced)
- 1 15-oz can kernel corn (drained)
- 1 15-oz can black beans (rinsed and drained)
- 1 tbsp granulated garlic
- 1 tbsp cumin
- ½ tsp cayenne pepper
- 4 cups water
- 2 tbsp lemon juice
- Salt/pepper to taste

INSTRUCTIONS

Place quinoa and water in medium pot over medium heat. Add a pinch of salt as it cooks. Bring to boil then reduce to a simmer, cover and let cook about 10 minutes.

Remove cover and stir. Place cover back on pot, turn heat to low, and allow to cook about 5 minutes or until water is cooked out. Remove from heat and allow to cool.

Once the quinoa is cooled, add the onion, tomato, black beans, and corn. Stir and add granulated garlic, cumin, cayenne pepper, lemon juice, and salt/pepper to taste. Stir ingredients again until mixed well.

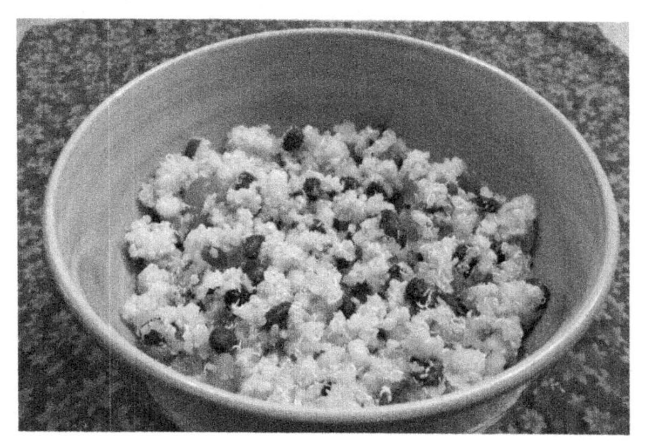

Place in refrigerator for about 30-45 minutes. Best served cold.

DESSERTS

BLUEBERRY MUFFINS

- 1 cup all-purpose whole wheat flour
- ½ cup all-purpose baking flour
- ½ cup rolled oats
- 1 tsp baking soda
- 1 tsp baking powder
- 2 tsp cinnamon
- 1 ⅛ tsp fast acting yeast (½ small pack)
- dash of salt
- ½ cup unsweetened almond milk
- 1 tbsp lemon juice
- ½ cup applesauce
- 1 flax egg (mix 1 tbsp ground flax and 3 tbsp water)
- 1 tsp vanilla extract
- ¼ cup maple syrup
- 2 tbsp molasses
- ½ cup fresh blueberries

INSTRUCTIONS

Mix lemon juice with almond milk and set aside. Mix all dry ingredients. In separate bowl mix all wet ingredients. Place wet ingredients in dry ingredients and mix well. Add blueberries. Place batter in muffin pan. Bake at 350 for about 20-30 minutes or until firm and golden brown.

Makes one dozen muffins.

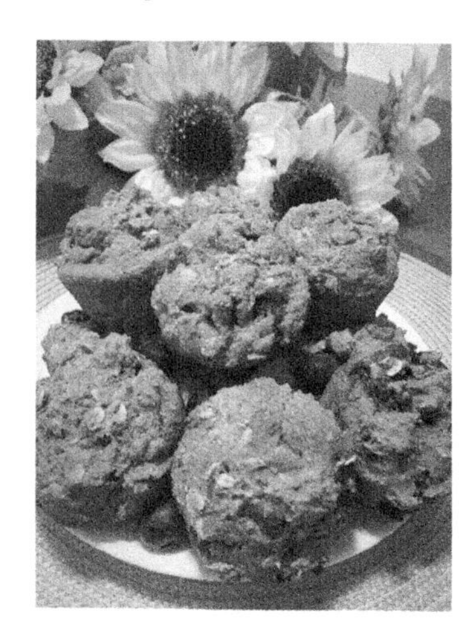

PUMPKIN BREAD

- 1 15-oz can pumpkin
- 2-3 over ripe bananas
- ¼ cup pure maple syrup
- ¼ cup molasses
- ¼ heaping cup of applesauce
- 2 flax eggs (2 tbsp ground flax and 6 tbsp water, whisked together)
- 1 tsp vanilla extract
- ¼ tsp almond extract
- 2 cups whole wheat pastry flour (Bob's Red Mill)
- ½ small packet of fast-acting yeast
- 1 tsp baking soda
- 1 tsp baking powder
- 1 tsp cinnamon
- dash of salt
- ⅓ cup non-dairy chocolate chips (optional)
- ⅓ cup chopped walnuts (optional)

INSTRUCTIONS

Pre-heat oven to 350° F (180° C).

Line bread pan with parchment paper.

Mix all wet ingredients (canned pumpkin to almond extract) in a bowl. Mix all dry ingredients (pastry flour to cinnamon) in a separate bowl.

Pour wet ingredients into dry ingredients and mix well. If adding the chocolate chips and walnuts, add them to the batter.

Pour the batter into the lined cake pan. Cook about 60-65 minutes. You can test by sticking a toothpick in bread: when it comes out clean, the pumpkin bread is done.

Banana Bread

- 4 over ripe bananas, mashed
- ¼ cup pure maple syrup
- ¼ cup molasses
- ¼ heaping cup of applesauce
- 2 flax eggs (2 tbsp ground flax and 6 tbsp water, whisked together)
- 1 tsp vanilla extract
- ¼ tsp almond extract
- 2 ½ cups whole wheat pastry flour (Bob's Red Mill)
- ½ small pack of fast-acting yeast
- 1 tsp baking soda
- 1 tsp baking powder
- 1 tsp cinnamon
- dash of salt
- ⅓ cup non-dairy chocolate chips (optional)
- ⅓ cup chopped walnuts (optional)

INSTRUCTIONS

Pre-heat oven to 350° F (180° C). Line bread pan with parchment paper.

Mix all wet ingredients (mashed bananas to almost extract) in a bowl. Mix all dry ingredients (pastry flour to salt) in a separate bowl. Pour wet ingredients into dry ingredients and mix well.

Pour wet ingredients into dry ingredients and mix well. If adding the chocolate chips and walnuts, add them to the batter.

Pour the batter into the lined cake pan. Cook about 60-65 minutes. You can test by sticking a toothpick in bread: when it comes out clean, the banana bread is done.

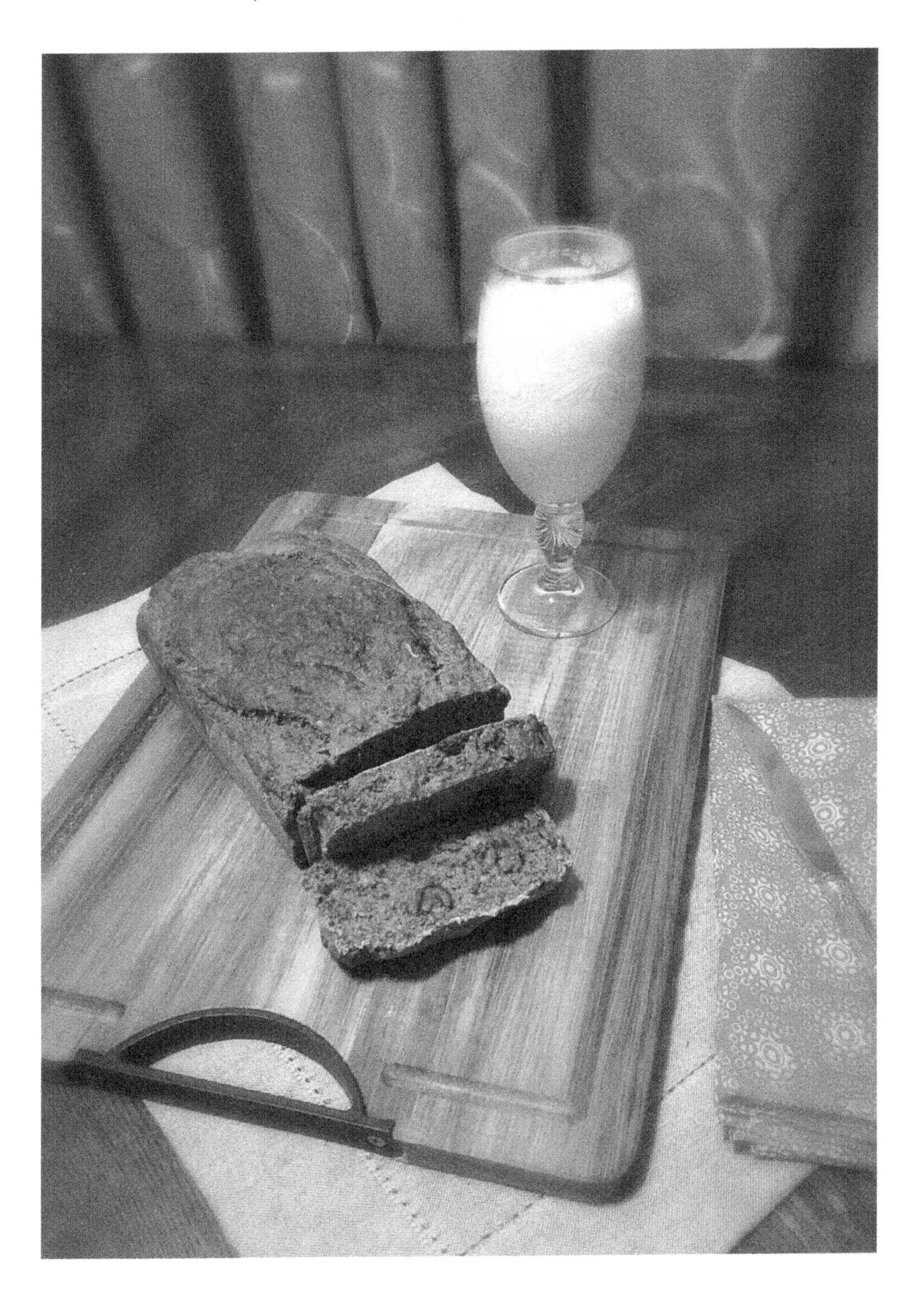

PECAN TART

- 1 ½ cups walnuts
- 18 pitted dates
- 2 tbsp raw organic sugar
- ½ cup firm tofu (not silken)
- ½ cup cashews (soaked in warm water about 30 minutes)
- 3 tbsp pure maple syrup
- ½ cup cashew milk
- 1 ½ cups chopped pecans
- ¼ cup non-dairy chocolate chips (optional)

INSTRUCTIONS

Pre-heat oven to 350° F (180° C).

CRUST: Place walnuts, 8 pitted dates, and organic sugar in food processor and blend until mixture is crumbly and begins to stick together. Place in pie pan, mashing it into the bottom and up the sides.

FILLING: Place 10 pitted dates, cashews (drained), tofu, maple syrup, and cashew milk into a food processor and blend. Pour into a bowl, and stir in the pecans and chocolate chips.

Pour into pie crust. Bake in oven until bubbly (about 30-45 minutes).

KIDDIE BITES

- 2 cups bite-size shredded wheat
- ¾ cup non-dairy chocolate chips
- ¼ to ½ cup organic powdered sugar

INSTRUCTIONS

Place shredded wheat in a large bowl that you can cover with a lid.

In a separate bowl place chocolate chips. Melt in microwave, watching carefully and checking often, until melted (about 1-2 minutes).

Pour melted chocolate chips over shredded wheat, put lid on the bowl, and shake well until evenly covered.

Open the lid and add the powdered sugar. Put the lid on and shake until evenly covered.

Pour out onto a cookie sheet and let set for about 1 hour. Place in an air tight container for storage.

Made in the USA
Monee, IL
04 March 2020

22705628R00031